For niece, Elisa – I hope you find this helpful with your food sensitivities.

Love you,
Auntie Sheryl

Cravings!

Your Guide to Freedom from the Agonizing Urge to Splurge

Sheryl Turgeon,
MPH, CHNC
**Integrative Health Coach
For Highly Sensitive Women**

www.SherylTurgeon.com
Your Health Potential, LLC

Copyright Notice

First Printing, 2016

ISBN-13: 978-1523411924

ISBN-10: 1523411929

Printed in the United States of America

Dedication

This book has been in me for quite a while, but it wouldn't have been completed and published without the encouragement and support of my wonderful coach, Laura West.

I also want to thank a fantastic editor, Elizabeth Cottrell, who gave me great suggestions in the writing of my first book.

Thank you, also, to my Business Manager Caroline Donnelly for her amazing technical assistance, without which this book would never have been published.

Last, but not least, I thank my husband, Paul, for his patience as I traveled to a cabin in Vermont to get this book off the ground. He's also given me support whether I'm writing and need a second pair of eyes, could use some design assistance, or just need him to fix dinner while I see a client. He's a true partner in every sense of the word.

Thank you all for being such bright lights in my life.

Contents

What Are Cravings & When Should You Worry?... 1

How Your Body Reacts to Sugar 5

My Story 11

Cravings Start from a Wounded Place..................... 17

How Feelings Create Cravings 23

An Amazing Client's Story... 27

How We Change... 29

BIG Food Preys on Our Instincts 33

How High Fructose Corn Syrup Hooks Us 35

What Connects Cravings and Food Sensitivities? .. 39

How We Develop Food Sensitivities 43

How's Your Digestion?.. 51

Enzymes for Better Digestion 59

Getting Off the Sugar Rollercoaster 63

What's Your Food-Mood Connection? 67

Self-Care Isn't Selfish 73

New Ways to Respond to Cravings 77

Healing from Cravings 81

Getting through the Crunch Times 87

Ways to Combat Social Pressure 89

What's in Your Future? A Case Study 95

Start Right Now: Freedom is Within Reach 101

Are You Ready to Take the First Step? 107

What Are Cravings and When Should You Worry?

Acraving, for this discussion, is an intense, urgent, and sometimes abnormal desire for specific foods or behavior. Cravings range from a desire for a piece of chocolate to compulsively downing a carton of ice cream.

We all get cravings at one time or another. Pregnant women are known for them. While I don't get many cravings anymore, if I eat something sweet, I need to watch myself, so that I don't start to eat more sugar the next day. If I'm not careful, I'll be off and running.

One nearly universal trigger of cravings is stress. We want to ease those anxious feelings with chips, sugar, shopping, carbohydrates, chocolate, alcohol—whatever is particularly soothing to us. When we start talking about substances such as cigarettes, alcohol, opiates, other drugs—or even sugar—we often speak in terms of addictions.

Basically, addiction occurs when the substance grows in its importance to you. First it becomes your "go to" whenever you're stressed, hungry, angry, lonely or tired. Soon it is an all-consuming craving that means more to you than anything else. You start to plan your life around it and basically, you find yourself having a love affair with the substance.

It can be a fine line between habit and addiction, so this book will cover those cravings that may teeter on the brink of addiction, but have not yet consumed your every waking thought.

Substance abuse may occur more rapidly with cigarettes, opiates, other drugs and alcohol requiring a deeper level of healing than I offer here, so please seek professional help if you suspect you have an addiction. For a self-test on addiction please visit:

https://ncadd.org/learn-about-alcohol/
alcohol-abuse-self-test.

I will talk about alcohol a bit, because it is a part of my story, and it may offer some valuable strategies; however, my goal is to help you understand why you get uncontrollable cravings and how to ease their grip through greater self-knowledge, better nutrition, better digestion, specific healing techniques, and deeper self-care leading to better moods.

Like many of my clients, you will get the right steps in the right order to help you heal and gain back control. Don't feel you must do everything at once though, or you will get stressed and want to revert to old behaviors. Take what works for you and practice adding that into your life. Then take another step. Before you know it, you'll be sailing into a cravings-free lifestyle!

Affirmation:
I am open to learning new ways to soothe my stress, from meditation to massage.

How Your Body Reacts To Sugar

Physiological processes can keep us hooked. If you start your day with coffee and a bagel, for instance, it is a set-up for sugar cravings, and here's why:

Both the caffeine and simple carbohydrates (i.e. bagel) shoot your blood sugar up like a roller coaster heading for the crest, and what goes up must come crashing down. If you add cream and sugar, you are spiking your blood sugar even more.

You might feel energized right after you eat, but a couple of hours later, your blood sugar drops below normal into the danger zone, and you feel anxious and irritable, ready to crash.

The body then senses a crisis and gives you signals to get more sugar fast. It is looking for a *quick fix,* because it sincerely needs glucose as fast as it can get it to climb out of the danger zone. If you had your breakfast around 8 a.m., by 10 or 10:30 you will crave something sweet or more carbohydrates like crackers, chips or an energy bar, because they act like sugar in your body.

Assuming you got the sugar you were craving; your body will be fine until lunch. Meanwhile, your blood sugar has already spiked and dipped twice—a cycle that leads to diabetes.

The yo-yo effect on your blood sugar has you in its grip at this point, so it doesn't take much to be persuaded to go to a fast-food restaurant for a heavy dose of more fat, salt, and sugar in the way of chicken nuggets, fries, or a shake.

You may even decide to be "good" and opt for the salad, if only the dressing weren't loaded with fat, salt, and sugar, too! Chances are you just sent your blood sugar up to the peak of the roller coaster again, so you are almost guaranteed to need another *quick fix*—like a candy bar—around 3 p.m.

Since all sorts of so-called healthy nutrition bars are available today, we can convince ourselves that the raisins, nuts, and seeds make the sugar, salt, and fat okay. Up goes the blood sugar again—just in time to keep us out of the danger zone once more.

In this typical scenario, let's say dinner is a bit late, since we have an extra report to get out or need to pick up the kids at soccer practice or we just want to unwind with some cheese and crackers and a glass of wine. In any case, we feel rushed when we do start cooking and rely on whatever short-cuts we can use to get the meal together fast.

We grab frozen veggies in their own special sauce or a box of pasta with cheese sauce that makes the fast food tastier. (By the way, they threw more fat, salt, and sugar into the sauce, so we wouldn't notice it would otherwise taste like cardboard!) We defrost some chicken breasts in the microwave and voilà! Dinner is served.

The cravings hit again full force a couple of hours later when the TV is blaring and every few minutes we see a food or pharmaceutical commercial. We just can't resist a few cookies from the cookie jar or that pint of ice cream that's calling to us from the freezer. We guiltily slink off to bed, thinking we'll do better tomorrow...

A client, Sarah, used to tell me she would eat an entire cake when she was overwhelmed by some difficult family problems. When she came to me, she reported it was almost like she went into a trance while she ate. Her behavior was always followed by guilt and remorse.

Together we gradually eliminated the sugar, while adding in fresh fruits and vegetables. We talked about other ways Sarah could de-stress and care for herself before she felt desperate enough to buy a cake.

After about five months, she dropped the extra weight and went down a couple of dress sizes. This was just in time for her high school reunion. She was thrilled that she had met her goal and told me everybody commented on how great she looked that night!

Whether it is bread, pastry, alcohol, chips, or a gooey dessert, sugar is sugar and sensitivity to it runs in families. We're going to take a look at why that is, as well as what to do about it if you're sugar sensitive and can't seem to leave it alone.

Cravings come in a variety of flavors, so if sugar isn't your thing, read on with your substance of choice in mind. If you routinely crave the same thing or a certain feeling always triggers the desire to escape, it's a signal (think flashing *yellow light*) that there's something more going on.

I hope sharing my own motivations, some physical chemistry, and pathways to change will help you gain some insight into what's going on for you.

Affirmation:
I am ready to release unhealthy habits that no longer serve me.

My Story

My grandfather used to say, "I only eat dinner to get to the dessert." My aunt is a self-confessed "chocoholic" and surreptitiously covets her pieces of dark chocolate every night. My mom was an alcoholic and died from the effects of the disease at 72. I have been in recovery for more than 25 years, myself.

I think my predisposition toward craving alcohol was activated the minute I took my first drink. I actually remember getting drunk and crying, which doesn't sound like much fun. The thing is, that didn't stop me, and alcohol soon became my friend in becoming more social and outgoing at parties.

A few glasses of wine *(which often ended up being a bottle)* relieved me after a long day at the office. I knew that I didn't just like alcohol, though. I'd had too many unintentional episodes where I ended up much more inebriated than I planned.

I was never certain how much I would drink or how drunk I would get. It's really an awful prison to both crave the substance and anguish over having too much of it. Other things in life become background music, and this play takes center stage.

It's really an awful prison to both crave the substance and anguish over having too much of it.

When I was 33 years old, I'd had enough. My decision wasn't prompted by a spectacular event. I had been attending *Alanon* meetings and seeing a counselor, as well as attending an *Adult Daughters of Alcoholics* group. I had danced around the subject for three years before I actually got to the point of putting the drink down.

Anyway, one night I had drunk a couple of glasses *(goblets)* of wine before going out with friends. They picked me up and we went to a bar. I remember drinking a couple of glasses of wine at the bar and not much else.

My friends took me home to my apartment and I evidently pulled the kitchen wastebasket out from under the sink before going to bed—was I preparing to vomit?

The next morning I felt sick. I had a terrible headache, and my whole body felt like it had been hit by a sledgehammer. That wasn't the worst part, though. It was how I felt inside—ashamed, frightened by the memory gaps, bone tired of the dance of wanting the substance, yet hating it.

That night some close friends were having a Memorial Day party and I had promised to be there, so I freshened up and drove the 10 minutes to their house.

They had made an alcoholic fruit punch, from which I immediately grabbed a glass, but it didn't make me feel any better. I still had that spacey, tired, sickly feeling. Usually, the "hair of the dog" got me back to normal, but not this night. I went home early and awoke Tuesday morning with the vow to quit drinking.

I had an appointment with my counselor that evening, so in preparation I went to a park across the street from my apartment and silently prayed for the strength to tell her I was an alcoholic. Going in to see her, I was *sweating bullets,* as they say. I dove right to the heart of the matter: "I'm an alcoholic and I'm going to quit drinking," I announced.

To my great surprise, she smiled, saying she knew and agreed that I should quit. We just needed to figure out when. I thought about my upcoming social plans for the summer—concerts to go to and parties to attend and said, "I'll quit in September." She firmly held me to my declaration, saying, "How about now?"

The rest, as they say, is history. Initially, all the feelings I had been stuffing down with alcohol came up in waves, and I felt like an emotional wreck. I remember calling my counselor and chastising her for not telling me what to expect.

It actually took me a year to attend *Alcoholics Anonymous* (AA) on a regular basis, but eventually I decided I wanted to enjoy people, places, and things, rather than shy away from them to stay sober, and I knew AA could help me do that.

Meanwhile, my mother's health was deteriorating, after having had two heart attacks and barely surviving with congestive heart failure. I went from my home in Massachusetts back to Michigan for a visit. During a quiet moment in the house, I told her about my struggle with alcohol and my newfound sobriety. "My God! I gave you that, too?" she exclaimed. I gently told her that it was her suffering with the disease that made me recognize it in myself at a stage when I could still quit.

Experiencing firsthand the ravages of my mother's and my own addiction inspired me to help other women to jump off the merry-go-round of self-hatred, denial, shame, and blame that seeps into our sense of self at every turn.

> *Helping women to thrive and live life to its fullest eventually became my passion and my career.*

If you or someone you know is experiencing the feelings I mentioned on some level, help is available. You can seek counseling from a therapist or help from an integrative health coach, who can help you on a physical, mental and emotional level to finally break free. (SherylTurgeon.com)

Life has opened up for me in ways I never thought possible before. The downward spiral that addictive behavior brings can be reversed, and recovery brings hope, action, freedom, and a new enthusiasm for living.

I finally moved out of my apartment in Walpole, MA, where I had lived for nine years waiting for *Mr. Right* to rescue me. I bought a condo on a lake and a dog, since I had come to terms with not having kids.

I developed the confidence to go back to school and earn a master's degree in public health. And I did meet *Mr. Right.* He was someone I never would have looked at twice (nor he at me) if I had been drinking.

Life is messy, and I have no magic bullets. What I have to share are personal stories and practical tools that will help regain your zest for living, finally free of the painful cycle that creates such physical and mental anguish.

Affirmation:
I embrace change, knowing it is for my highest good.

Cravings Start from
A Wounded Place

The main problem with addiction is when you're in its grip, you can't imagine life without the substance or crutch, yet it is exactly this crutch that is keeping you in pain. I think cravings start from a wounded place too.

When we experience cravings, we want something—love, comfort, attention, affection—and we are unable to get it. We reach for a substitute *(name your poison)* and find it eases those painful feelings of lack and emptiness. We soon learn to reach only for the substitute. It's safer and always provides satisfaction, or so we think.

Kelly was a client who had so much going for her. She was advancing in her career and seemed super capable, managing any task handed to her—even if it meant working all weekend.

Boundaries were an issue for Kelly, though. She would run herself ragged, until she developed an illness that forced her to take time out. Comfort foods like pasta, bread, and pastries were her "quick fix" for feeling overwhelmed.

When we started coaching together, we talked about her goals to eat healthy and lose some weight. She was a smart woman and loved what she learned about trying new whole foods and how they react in the body. But she wasn't going to meet her goals until she started to say "no."

Kelly began to add in time to enjoy shopping for and preparing good, fresh food. She found a way to move that she enjoyed. She scheduled some time for fun with her husband and friends. She learned to tell family members and her employer she was not available sometimes.

Kelly thrived with her new approach to life. She did drop weight and felt much healthier, but realized her transformation went much deeper. She began to honor herself in a way she never had before and that was even more valuable to her than dropping 48 pounds!

Unfortunately, when it comes to cravings, we can't really fool ourselves deep down. We know when we still haven't fulfilled our elemental needs and as hard or as often as we try to substitute our way to happiness, it just doesn't happen. In fact, the reverse is usually true. We spiral downward to a greater and greater need for the substance/behavior, because the glaring fact is *we are not happy.*

From this vantage point, the idea of letting go of the substance is ludicrous. "What? Give up the only thing easing my pain?"

I found it necessary to dig down to access a hope more powerful than what I could muster myself... I had to open my heart to believe in others who had gone before me. I borrowed their hope until I could find my own because all I felt at first was pain.

But after ripping off the band-aid of alcohol, my hope that life could get better grew and my ability to appreciate some of the more subtle aspects of living resurfaced—aspects I thought had gone by the wayside.

I remember driving down the road in Walpole, MA, on a sunny autumn day and literally falling in love with the sparkling sunshine through the trees, the birds chirping, and the peace I felt inside.

In AA, they call this renewed appreciation a "Pink Cloud." All I know is this: Life began to look a whole lot better than it had in years!

I can't say that magically, everything that was "wrong" in my life suddenly disappeared. I did discover a genuine fondness for being alive that spurred me onward to address issues I previously only complained about and had drunk over.

We resist change out of fear, and if you're going to break through to freedom, I want to assure you that it is well worth the effort!

When I was willing to shift my perspective and open up to a different way of being in the world, new opportunities opened up. I want to share that with you, because tackling cravings takes courage. You need all the support and encouragement you can get. We resist change out of fear, and if you're going to break through to freedom, I want to assure you that it is well worth the effort!

Just to acknowledge what we're up against, my instructor and the founder of the Institute for Integrative Nutrition, Joshua Rosenthal, used to say people would rather change their religion than change their eating habits.

I want to add that cravings happen on many levels from emotional to physiological to spiritual. We need to shed some light on what those aspects are all about, because awareness is the first step in changing a behavior—and I know you wouldn't be reading this if you didn't want to make that change.

Affirmation:
Fear is False Evidence
Appearing Real.
LOVE Triumphs over FEAR.

How Feelings Create Cravings

What do you crave? The typical cravings are for sugar, salt, fat, caffeine, or alcohol (a form of sugar). The key is getting at the feelings that are associated with the cravings before, during, and after consumption.

How did you feel before that first bite or sip? What happens when you eat that food or consume that substance? Do you experience feelings of warmth, comfort, euphoria or confidence?

If you want to release the behavior, you must decipher the craving and address the need first.

Your clue to what you are seeking is in those feelings. You can start to journal about your relationship with the craving and let your mind wander to where you are missing those emotions in your life. You can begin by downloading my Awareness Journal (sherylturgeon.com/cravings-your-guide-to-freedom/cravings-bonuses) that helps you track your feelings quickly by simply filling in the blanks.

If you want to release the behavior, you must decipher the craving and address the need first.

I help my clients do this is with a tool I call their *Spheres of Influence*™. It helps us determine where their levels of satisfaction are in every aspect of their life and focus on how to bring in more joy and happiness to each area of need.

We human beings are pretty amazing and complex. Nothing we do is without reason. In fact, I often say to my clients that *the craving is the solution—not the problem.*

We all want to feel joyous and free. Renowned author and inspirational speaker, the late Wayne Dyer, PhD, said feeling good is akin to feeling God. In our essence, our natural state is infinitely loving and abundantly joyful. Everything we do, however misguided it may be, is an attempt to get back to that natural state.

Now think of the various behaviors we develop in response to life's pain, frustrations, and disappointments. On every level of our being, the need to change the behavior must become more attractive than the need to continue it. If it is serving a purpose and we don't find another way to meet that need, we're stuck with the craving.

A word of caution here—on your journey to becoming free of cravings and compulsive behaviors, just remember we're all human and we don't often do it perfectly right away.

You may slip here and there until you can ingrain the new behaviors into your habitual responses. This is where your compassion for yourself comes in. **YOU MUST FORGIVE YOURSELF FOR ANY SLIPS**. Not everyone has them, but if you do, just move on.

I can't begin to stress how important this is. It is the condemning feelings that lead us right back into the same old behavioral pattern we're learning to change.

Treat a slip as a learning situation. A baby learning to walk doesn't give up after the first try. She is at it again and again and again until she gets it. There is no ego involved—just a willingness to keep trying. This mindset will take you where you want to go.

Many of us have the old tapes playing in our heads—the ones from parents or others close to us who often criticized, blamed, or shamed us. We no longer need that outside voice, since it has become a part of our own critical voice. Keep an eye out for it and answer it with an affirmation.

I have several affirmations you can choose from to stick on your refrigerator or place by your bedside to read as you start your day. You can download the ones you want and then come back for more here: sherylturgeon.com/cravings-your-guide-to-freedom/cravings-bonuses

It may take some therapy or coaching to quiet the voice and replace it with patience, love and compassion until you can give it to yourself. Learning to play new tapes confirming your self-worth is one of the keys to success in overcoming unhealthy cravings, and I'm passionate about helping you do that!

Affirmation:
I deserve love and compassion whether I succeed or start over.

An Amazing Client's Story

Dianna came from an over-protective, critical family. She had grown up in an insulated environment. Her innocence was the first thing that struck me when we met. She had used lap-band surgery to shed a few hundred extra pounds, but she didn't know how to eat well. We set out to change that.

I realized in our sessions that Dianna needed the support to speak on her own behalf and feel empowered to take control of her life. Food had been her only outlet for feelings she felt powerless to change. We gently journeyed forward in terms of establishing new eating habits and helping Dianna find her voice.

During our coaching together, this 30-something woman learned to drive and got her license. She created her own business, tapping into her amazing sensitive traits and unique abilities. She dropped more weight and loved how much better she felt. Dianna was well on her way to creating a new life that supported her and expressed her beautiful soul.

Affirmation:
The journey toward my goals gets easier with each step.

How We Change

Renowned author and physician Christiane Northrup, MD, once said she pictures her negative voice on her left shoulder and her positive voice on her right. When the negative voice speaks up, she acknowledges that it is trying to protect her and thanks it. Then she clearly and firmly tells it what she is going to do from the right shoulder.

My efforts to resolve my own drinking issues were much more strategic than I was aware of on a conscious level. I had put into place many social supports in terms of groups, a counselor, and education about what it was doing to me.

Deep down, I knew the gig was up, and I had drawn to me the people who could help me long before I sat down in that park to pray.

Another key factor was that I chose surrender instead of control in confronting my craving.

I chose surrender instead of control in confronting my craving.

Geneen Roth, author of *Breaking Free from Emotional Eating,* describes the process as letting go of your side of the rope in a tug of war. When you let go, there is no more war. The rope just goes limp. That is where we want to be to loosen the grip of our cravings on us.

I turned over my struggle to the Universe/God/Source and asked for help. While I don't consider myself religious, I am spiritual and I believe we are all connected to something greater than ourselves.

It is this power that I tapped into sitting on a park bench over 25 years ago. And this power enabled me to step off of the merry-go-round of my addictive behavior. I asked and I was answered by this power in a divinely simple manner that can still bring tears of gratitude to my eyes.

Getting ready for change may be a conscious or unconscious process. When we reach the point where we make a phone call or respond to an email, we're ready. We may be tired of the endless struggle. We may be forewarned of impending illness. We may just reach a point where we know we can feel better and are ready to take action.

The point is we're ready to put down what doesn't work and pick up what does. My ideal clients are actively looking for a solution. They come to me to get relief from cravings and realize they need to change their habits or patterns to have more of a choice in how they live their lives.

- It takes commitment.
- It takes the willingness to reach out for help.
- It takes the courage to change.

I know first-hand that it's hard to do it alone. I also know that when we have the support of someone who is our champion and understands our struggles, we can quit falling into the same old trap.

My clients have made changes that transformed their lives and so can you. The first step is committing to do what it takes to get better. After that, you need to get in touch with someone who can help you. (SherylTurgeon.com) You will be amazed at how fantastic it feels when the cravings are gone and you are free from struggle!

Affirmation:
I'm ready to put down what doesn't work and pick up what does.

BIG Food Preys
On Our Instincts

T*he End of Overeating* by Michael Kessler, MD, pulls back the curtain on how the food industry has preyed upon our natural desires for fat, salt, and sugar to sell us processed foods that are loaded with the stuff. As the competition grew, so did the amounts of sugar, fat and salt.

What that does to our bodies, besides making us fat, is interfere with the production of two hormones called ghrelin and leptin. These hormones are designed to tell us when we are hungry and when we are full, but they stop working when we eat foods that overload us with more fat, salt, and sugar than our bodies were meant to handle.

Someone once compared this interference to whispering to a friend at a rock concert—you'll never hear them, just as we stop hearing our hormones speak to us when we are blasted with too much fat, salt, and sugar.

Another major player in the physiologically addictive cycle is high fructose corn syrup (HFCS). Despite what the corn manufacturers would have you believe, HFCS has to be the single most damaging and addictive sweetener conjured up during the last century.

Overconsumption of sugar is at the root of many serious chronic conditions, but HFCS enhances those destructive qualities and does the job faster.

Since HFCS was introduced in processed foods like ketchup, cookies, and, most notably, soda in the 1970s, the average American's consumption rose from zero to 60 pounds per person per year.

At the same time, obesity rates tripled and diabetes rates increased seven-fold as noted by *UltraMetabolism* Author Mark Hyman, MD.

Affirmation: I am an independent thinker who takes care of my body using my intuition.

How High Fructose Corn Syrup Hooks Us

L et's briefly take a look at how both sucrose and fructose are metabolized in the body to discover how this is affecting us. Derived from beets and sugar cane, sucrose is made up of 50 percent glucose and 50 percent fructose.

These are simple sugars that are metabolized differently in the body. When we consume glucose, blood sugar levels rise. The pancreas releases insulin to absorb the glucose from the bloodstream and delivers it to the cells for energy.

Fructose, as in high fructose corn syrup, goes directly to the liver. No digestion is required, so it is more rapidly absorbed by the bloodstream. Fructose triggers the liver to produce fats like triglycerides and cholesterol and is a major cause of a fatty and damaged liver (Once seen only in advanced-stage alcoholics, it now affects 70 million people—including children!)

Too much glucose and fructose leads to metabolic imbalances that increase appetite and weight gain and contribute to diabetes, heart disease, dementia, osteoporosis, arthritis, cancer, Alzheimer's disease, and more.

But fructose in fruit and fructose in processed foods don't act on the body in the same way. Naturally occurring fructose stays within a 50/50 ratio of fructose to glucose, and the body's absorption is slowed by the fruit's fiber, so the body is able to metabolize it properly.

Fructose in HFCS, however, has a 55/45 ratio of fructose to glucose, so it requires more energy to be absorbed by the gut, causing it to soak up more Adenosine Triphosphate or ATP (our cells' energy source). The effect of this depletion of energy in our gut then causes deterioration of the lining of our intestines.

"High doses of HFCS have been proven to literally punch holes in the intestinal lining, allowing nasty byproducts of toxic gut bacteria and partially digested food proteins to enter the bloodstream and trigger inflammation," says Dr. Hyman. This process underlies body-wide inflammation, chronic disease, and accelerated aging.

A great DVD called **King Corn** (https://youtu.be/tGSsScjwQ3Y) by a couple of Massachusetts Institute of Technology (MIT) graduates brings home the obsequious use of HFCS. They are on a road trip after graduating from school, and they stop to see their buddy, a research scientist, who analyzes their hair.

To their shock and dismay, they find they are made up of 97 percent corn! They had been stopping at fast food eateries on the road, and most of that food contains—you guessed it—high fructose corn syrup!

At the risk of giving away too much of the storyline, they decide to grow their own acre of corn and follow it through to delivery and consumption in New York City.

A conversation with a soda-drinking, diabetic New York cab driver and a quick stop at a convenience store where every product contains HFCS illustrate how thoroughly this one product has infiltrated and created havoc in our lives.

Affirmation:
I am committed to giving my body the best nourishment available.

What Connects Cravings And Food Sensitivities?

Food sensitivities and cravings have a peculiar relationship that we need to explore. Our digestive systems often stop working properly after years of consuming processed foods, drugs (especially antibiotics and Nonsteroidal anti-inflammatory drugs (NSAIDs)), sugar, HFCS, and other toxins).

Food allergies and sensitivities may result, in which symptoms develop from ingesting certain foods.

I used to love garlic and onions! If I was cooking, you could bet they were among the ingredients. Over time, I developed headaches with greater frequency and intensity.

A bizarre episode occurred several years ago when I flew to a National

Community Health Center Conference in Washington, D.C.

At the time, I was CEO of a federally-funded community health center and routinely attended the bi-annual federal conference. Luckily, this year I brought the Center's nursing director with me.

We met for dinner in the hotel restaurant our first night, where I ate a burger with onions and fries. We left the restaurant early to return to our rooms, as we had a full day ahead of us.

In the wee hours of the morning, I found myself standing over the bed rummaging through my conference materials. I was frantically trying to figure out where I was! It seems I had developed transient global amnesia.

This condition occurs perhaps once in a lifetime and affects 3.4 to 5.2 people per 100,000 per year. When 7:30 a.m. rolled around, the nursing director called me to join her for breakfast. But judging by my confused state over the phone, she quickly concluded I needed help.

She came to my room to see what was happening, and I kept repeating myself. I did remember I was married and had continually punched my home phone number on my cell phone trying to reach my husband, who was already at work. The poor man had numerous frantic messages on the answering machine that he'll never forget.

Meanwhile, the hotel doctor came up to assess me and recommended that I go to the Emergency Room of University Hospital.

I received CT scans and a spinal tap as they tried to figure out what was wrong with me. As time went on, the nursing director was able to reach my husband. Both he and my sister decided to hop on the next flight to Washington, DC.

By evening, the amnesia was subsiding. Unfortunately, the residents involved in my care never mentioned that I shouldn't sit up or walk around after a spinal.

I insisted on meeting with our federal grant officer the next day, so we had booked a flight home a bit later.

I knew that if I didn't start listening to my body's signs of stress and distress, I might not bounce back the next time.

It was in the airport that I developed the mother of all migraines. My sister and husband debated about whether or not I should fly. However, I managed to get on the plane and made it back to Massachusetts safely.

After that incident, I seemed to get migraines on a regular basis and you know what the main culprits were that triggered them? Onions and garlic! The last thing I ate before the episode.

My body had become chemically imbalanced from a lifetime of ingesting sugar, foods to which I was sensitive, and other toxic substances in the environment.

It was evident that this was a major warning signal and I knew that if I didn't start listening to my body's signs of stress and distress, I might not bounce back the next time.

Affirmation:
My health is my priority, even if it means saying "no" to someone.

How We Develop Food Sensitivities

Food sensitivities develop when a food molecule leaks outside the single-celled wall of the intestines and is seen by the body as an invader. Phagocytes (white blood cells that protect the body by ingesting harmful foreign particles) go in for the attack, and antibodies develop against that food.

Consequently, the next time the food is consumed, the body still sees it as a foreign invader and continues to mount a defense, whether the food actually leaks outside of the intestinal wall or not. The more often we eat a particular food, the more likely it is to become *the enemy.*

With the right diet and healing protocols, though, clients who have been afraid to eat all but a handful of foods have been able to turn around their sensitivities and enjoy a variety of meals.

We vacillate between feeling okay and lousy, and we assume most people feel this way—not true!

People with food sensitivities may or may not be aware of them, although most who seek help do so because of symptoms that might include recurring headaches or migraines, irritable bowel syndrome, abdominal pain, recurrent bladder infections, chronic muscle pain, poor memory, sinus conditions, insomnia, depression, fuzzy thinking, constipation, gas, indigestion, bloating, mood swings, aggressive behavior, nervousness, anxiety, skin rashes, and shortness of breath.

Many of us with food sensitivities don't really know what it is like to feel well. We vacillate between feeling okay and lousy, and we assume most people feel this way—not true!

It's quite possible to heal and feel vibrant and alive by feeding your body whole, fresh foods that reduce inflammation and support it, eliminating sugar and processed foods, and creating balance in your physical and emotional environment.

It seems that high sensitivity in one area of the body often correlates with an overall higher sensitivity throughout the nervous system. This can actually be an advantage, because if you have a sensitive nature, it will guide you once you start listening to it.

As a coach for Highly Sensitive Women, I have helped women tap into their gifts of sensitivity to guide them to greater health, happiness and success.

One of my highly sensitive clients, Jennifer, was down to only a handful of foods when she started coaching with me. She had the telltale circles under her eyes, along with bloating, pain, and irritable bowel. She had been to physicians but wasn't getting any better.

We used food sensitivity testing and discovered her food sensitivities were through the roof! It was a six-month process to regain her health, as we eliminated all the foods that were causing inflammation and added in foods that could help her heal.

It isn't easy to give up the foods you love, and Jennifer's commitment to the process was awesome!

While we were able to offer substitutes for many of the foods she enjoyed, if she had just one bite of a food she was sensitive to, her antibodies would be reactivated and she would need to go back to day one in the elimination process.

Her desire to get better was stronger than her desire for inflammatory foods, though, and she stuck to her plan. Jennifer now eats a wide variety of foods—especially the seafood she once loved but made her sick!

The body tends to crave the food to which it has developed an allergy.

If you suspect you have food sensitivities, tests are available to reveal which foods are causing problems. I use tests such as the ELISA/ACT lab test with clients to detect the IgG antibodies present in their bloodstream.

Depending on the level of antibodies, sensitivities to specific foods will be rated as moderate or severe in terms of response. A protocol for avoidance is recommended based on that analysis, ranging from three to six months.

The key is removing the food long enough for the antibodies you have built up to die off. We also introduce nourishing, anti-inflammatory foods and support your healing with targeted micronutrient supplements.

Researchers found a curious result of the food sensitivity process and one that is counterproductive: The body tends to crave the food to which it has developed an allergy.

One explanation is the body is no longer getting the nutrients it needs from that food. I get the image of our digestive system crying out to us, "Hit me again, I know I can get it right this time!"

Another reason for the phenomenon is that it is actually a stage in the disease process. When the immune system is exhausted, as it is when we repeatedly eat foods that leak through our intestinal wall, we get a reaction like those listed earlier.

If we continue to eat the same foods, the body adapts to the irritant. The phagocytes weaken, and a more chronic reaction develops, taking the body longer to return to balance.

This phenomenon is similar to the process of smoking cigarettes. At first, we cough and may even vomit after smoking. Soon, though, our bodies learn to adapt to the tar and nicotine to the point where we develop withdrawal symptoms when we stop smoking.

The body's resistance has diminished, and the alarm reaction disappears. It is at this stage of adaptation that we can become addicted to the substance.

We develop withdrawal symptoms whenever we are not eating that food or drinking that drink, because the body has learned to chemically change once it's been ingested.

It usually takes five to 10 days for withdrawal symptoms to disappear. But eating certain foods and taking the right supplements will help alleviate the symptoms.

A word of caution though—if instead we continue to consume the substance, degenerative disease is likely to follow.

Affirmation:
My awareness of how food affects
my body grows stronger every day.
I use my awareness to treat
my body well.

How's Your Digestion?

When our digestion isn't working properly, the body will often crave salt as a way of obtaining minerals it lacks.

According to Nancy Appleton, author of *Suicide by Sugar,* "No mineral is an island. Minerals can only function in relation to each other. If one mineral drops in the bloodstream, the other minerals will not function as well... and the body's chemistry is thrown off."

Even a small change in mineral composition can have a powerful effect on the body. Digestive enzymes, for example, need minerals to function properly. When the enzymes aren't functioning well because of a deficiency in minerals, not all of the food is digested and broken down adequately.

Dr. William Philpott, in his book *Brain Allergies,* explains that improper digestion of proteins creates unusable protein molecules that are absorbed into the blood, reaching body tissues in their partially digested form (a condition referred to as *Leaky Gut*).

The body sees the undigested food as invasive, which can cause toxicity and inflammation in various organs or tissues within the body.

The tiny, partially digested food particles create different chronic conditions, depending on where the bloodstream deposits them.

When they go to the joints, they can cause arthritis. According to Philpott, when they go into the skin, they can cause hives, psoriasis or eczema, and when they inflame the lining of the digestive tract, colon or rectum, they can cause ulcerative colitis, irritable bowel syndrome or Crohn's disease.

White blood cells need a regular supply of properly digested protein to bring the body back into homeostasis. Unfortunately, stress, sugar, food sensitivities, drugs, *Candida,* and other factors keep suppressing the immune system, so that it becomes less able to regulate itself.

Leaky Gut Syndrome is pervasive in today's environment. Chronic or prolonged stress changes the immune system's ability to respond quickly and affects our ability to heal, reducing our IgA antibodies (the immune system's first line of defense) and DHEA (dehydroepiandrosterone, an adrenal hormone that reduces aging and stress). Digestion slows down and toxic metabolites increase.

Alcohol, sugar, birth control pills, and stress can all lead to Leaky Gut. An imbalance in our intestines called dysbiosis results because parasites, Candida and other bacterial organisms start to flourish. They get into our intestinal wall and break down the brush borders or cilia lining the intestines.

Antibiotics, NSAIDs, and other medications used over a long period of time can lead to Leaky Gut as well. Antibiotics kill off both the friendly and unfriendly bacteria, upsetting the delicate balance in our intestines. Without the proper probiotics to replenish the friendly bacteria, Candida is likely to take hold.

Environmental contaminants, over-consumption of alcohol, and poor food choices (processed foods) are also important pieces of the puzzle in Leaky Gut. Each contributing factor puts a strain on the liver, which then allows toxins into the blood stream.

> ***Leaky Gut is not a small annoyance, but an important warning sign that you could be on a pathway toward serious disease.***

When antibodies have built up over a long period of time, the liver becomes overwhelmed and can't eliminate food antigens. That is when the antigens enter the blood stream and trigger a delayed sensitivity response, inflammation, cell damage, and disease.

This means Leaky Gut is not a small annoyance, but an important warning sign that you could be on a pathway toward serious disease.

Asthma, eczema, fibromyalgia, food allergies, chronic sinusitis, irritable bowel, urticaria, migraine, fungal disorders, and inflammatory joint disorders, such as rheumatoid arthritis, have been associated with Leaky Gut Syndrome.

Research shows that Leaky Gut Syndrome is almost always connected to autoimmune diseases such as Crohn's, Lupus Erythematosus, Multiple Sclerosis, Thyroiditis or Chronic Fatigue Syndrome.

Once the intestinal tract is damaged, free radicals and inflammation result, worsening Leaky Gut. Nutrients like Vitamins E and C, selenium, zinc, l-glutamine, and Coenzyme Q10 will help cells regenerate and support the healing process.

In summary, people with food sensitivities aren't metabolizing their foods properly and therefore have a greater need for pure, hypoallergenic nutritional supplementation. Eating whole, fresh foods, getting regular exercise, and managing stress with intuitive self-care will support your healing process.

I remember a couple who came to me with skin rashes. As we discussed their symptoms and diet, I was almost certain we were dealing with an imbalance in their digestive bacteria.

We went through a *Candida* questionnaire, and both scored high on the indicator for this overgrowth of harmful bacteria. They needed to cut out sugar and yeast, as well as adding in lots of fresh whole foods and probiotics.

Gradually, over a three-month period, their rashes disappeared, along with other irritating chronic symptoms. Now they know the protocol if their digestive bacteria ever gets out of balance again. Sometimes, the cure is pretty simple.

You can find additional digestive support from probiotics in foods like kefir and yogurt or, if you are sensitive to dairy, try home-made sauerkraut or pickles. Essentially, probiotics replenish the healthy bacteria that keep our system in balance.

Be careful as you introduce probiotics into your system, as die-off from the bad bacteria is likely to occur.

Too much die-off means greater symptoms of illness, so start with one teaspoon of your probiotic food or a couple of supplements per day. To help you safely and comfortably begin your recovery, pay attention to how you feel and report any problems to your health care professional.

Affirmation:
I am whole and in balance.
All systems in my body function
in harmony.

Enzymes for Better Digestion

Enzymes can increase the digestibility and accessibility of proteins and carbohydrates in the small intestine. As we age and consume processed foods, medications and even cooked foods, we continually draw on our pancreatic enzymes to metabolize our food.

We end up with fewer and fewer enzymes to support the body. Adding effective enzyme support from raw foods and the right supplements helps to strengthen our bodies and promotes healing from food sensitivities.

Herbs and spices also play an amazing role in regaining digestive health. For example, cumin is thought to stimulate the secretion of enzymes from the pancreas, which can then help us absorb nutrients. Oregano has strong antiviral, antibacterial, and anti-parasitic properties that aide digestion and strengthen the immune system. Other important spices include thyme, cinnamon, and turmeric.

Thomas Rau, MD, author of *The Swiss Guide to Optimum Health,* spells out four tips for avoiding dietary allergic reactions:

- Pay attention to unexplained malaise and other undiagnosed symptoms. See if there is any correlation between how you feel and what you eat.
- Rotate what you eat. Aside from providing all the nutrients you need, a variety of foods protects against repeated contact with any food allergen.
- Avoid processed foods, genetically engineered crops, and artificial ingredients, which can trigger severe allergic reactions.
- Notice when you develop a compulsive craving and consider it a warning sign.

Affirmation:
I treat cravings as a warning that
something is out of balance.
I get the help I need to release the
craving and create balance in my
body, mind and spirit.

Getting Off the Sugar Rollercoaster

The body still does an amazing job of processing nearly everything we put in it, including sugar. Since refined sugar is stripped of all nutrients, the body uses its own supply to absorb it. When we eat sugar, we lose nutrients we need, like B vitamins, calcium, phosphorus, and iron.

Sugar basically has a siphoning effect that can create a gnawing hunger for whatever elements are missing from our bodies, from fiber and vitamins to minerals and protein. The result can be bingeing behavior, according to Anne Marie Colbin, author of *Food and Healing.*

Dr. Roger Williams created a nutritional protocol for alcoholism, which works equally well to relieve sugar addiction and replaces many of the lost vitamins and minerals.

The cornerstone of his treatment is large quantities of B-complex vitamins, along with chromium, vitamin C, lecithin, L-glutamine, and a vegetable-rich, complex carbohydrate diet.

Another vital step in regaining balance is to eat a nutritious breakfast that supplies enough protein and complex carbohydrates in order to jump-start your metabolism.

Eating small healthy snacks every few hours helps too, by keeping the blood sugar steady. Specific snacks are included in your bonus resources, which you can access on my website: sherylturgeon.com/cravings-your-guide-to-freedom/cravings-bonuses.

But changing your eating patterns doesn't happen overnight. In fact, attempting to change in dramatic ways usually backfires, as evidenced by the endless diets so many of us have tried.

I recommend substituting one healthier version of the food you crave at a time, along with introducing the appropriate supplements. As you start down the path to feeling better, you'll begin to slip out of the grip of that nagging urge to splurge.

Affirmation:
Slower is best in the long run.
I'm getting better one step
at a time.

What's Your Food-Mood Connection?

We wouldn't have difficulty with cravings if there weren't a food-mood connection. As individuals, our sensitivity to that connection varies, from moderate to intense.

Kathleen Des Maisons, author of *Potatoes Not Prozac,* explains what happens in the brain when sugar-sensitive people eat sweets and simple carbohydrates or drink alcohol. Three internal factors influence our cravings for sweets:

1. Des Maisons says that we naturally have low serotonin, a neurotransmitter in the brain that creates a sense of relaxation and peace.

It also influences impulse control and the ability to plan ahead. Low serotonin results in the tendency to be depressed, impulsive, scattered, to overreact, and to crave sweets (which temporarily raise the level of serotonin).

2. Another piece of the brain puzzle is called beta-endorphin, a chemical that can either drive you toward addiction or lift your spirits. When the body experiences pain, it releases beta-endorphin, such as when a long-distance runner feels "high" after a 10-mile sprint.

Low beta-endorphin results in feelings of tearfulness, low self-esteem, being easily overwhelmed, depressed, and having a low tolerance for pain. You also crave sugar. Sounds like feelings experienced by a lot of highly sensitive people, doesn't it? Maybe there is something to that runner's high...

3. The third influencing factor is our blood sugar. As I mentioned earlier, when it rises and dips like a rollercoaster, our emotions do the same.

The brain requires a steady supply of glucose to feel good. If your blood sugar level is too low, you're likely to feel tired all the time, restless, confused, easily frustrated, irritable, and have difficulty with memory and concentration. This condition is known as hypoglycemia and is often a precursor to diabetes.

When your imbalanced body chemistry is sugar sensitive, you get a bigger "hit" every time you consume sugar, alcohol, or simple carbohydrates.

If feelings like these frequently influence your behavior, it is a good indication that your body is out of balance. Here's the hook: When your imbalanced body chemistry is sugar sensitive, you get a bigger "hit" every time you consume sugar, alcohol, or simple carbohydrates.

That makes a steady diet of the sweet stuff very attractive, which also keeps your moods fluctuating up and down and, as we learned earlier, takes its toll on the immune system.

How do serotonin, beta-endorphin and glucose levels in your body interact?

When you ingest even a small amount of sugar, you want more because of a mechanism in the beta-endorphin system called priming. In order to put a halt to that craving mechanism, you need to eliminate sugar from your diet and balance your brain chemistry.

Even after you have stopped consuming sugar for a while, you are at risk for priming. Your brain compensates for a naturally low level of beta-endorphin and serotonin by creating more neurotransmitter receptors to soak up the amounts you do have.

If you eliminate the substances that have been charging up your brain chemicals, you create more receptors. The next time you eat or drink that substance, you get an even bigger "hit," causing greater euphoria. It is only natural that you would want to repeat that experience, and you're off on your rollercoaster once more.

Dr. Des Maisons developed a food plan designed to boost tryptophan in the brain as a means of increasing serotonin. The idea is if you eat a protein like turkey, and follow it with a complex carbohydrate such as a potato, it will give tryptophan the boost it needs to cross the blood-brain barrier and increase your serotonin.

I have found that using a whole life approach to boost my serotonin and regain my balance works best for me. When detoxifying from sugar, I recommend my clients do several things that feel good and boost serotonin, from a trip to the beach to a walk in the park to quiet meditation or even great sex.

Eliminating the substances that are aggravating your system often causes withdrawal symptoms that can be eased with a detoxifying bath, exercise, meditation, or pleasurable music. It is a time to be gentle with yourself and draw on the support of friends and family.

Incidentally, Michael Ellsberg, who wrote an article in *Forbes Magazine,* "How I Overcame Bipolar II," discovered a connection between sugar, refined carbohydrates, alcohol, and coffee when it came to his manic and depressive episodes.

As a last-ditch effort to heal, he refrained from coffee, alcohol, and sugar for a year. He went from being penniless and suicidal to regaining economic and emotional stability and enjoying a loving, happy marriage. He says his occasional indulgences since then have not derailed his empowering new lifestyle.

Affirmation:
I enjoy life's sweetness without sugar. I think more clearly, have better moods and feel more energetic now.

Self-Care Isn't Selfish

The Art of Extreme Self Care by Cheryl Richardson opened my eyes to the beneficial effects of nurturing yourself well. We can't give what we haven't got, so giving until we are exhausted doesn't do us or anyone else any good.

Yet, many of us have learned to put ourselves last and we wind up resentful, in need of what I call the *quick fix*. We are at our wits' end emotionally and use food (usually sweets) or alcohol to pacify ourselves. Does this sound familiar?

The idea was really brought home to me when I was commuting from Providence, RI, to New York City each month to the Institute for Integrative Nutrition, working full time as CEO of a community health center and managing a household with my husband, three step-children, and two dogs.

Caring for ourselves runs much deeper than what might be considered selfish. It means honoring ourselves in a way that reflects who we are inside.

I was talking with my coach about how tired I was, while planning a big Easter dinner for our extended family. She said, "What do you think your family would rather have—an exhausted woman who has everything on the table but can't carry on a conversation, or a mother who postpones this until she can find pleasure in it and be present? I finally got it. Taking care of myself was beneficial to everybody!

Caring for ourselves runs much deeper than what might be considered selfish. It means honoring ourselves in a way that reflects who we are inside. This is especially important and usually difficult for most women.

We have often been raised to feel guilty about taking care of our own needs for alone time, quiet, rest, or other balancing behaviors. Yet, learning to listen to what we need and following through on it is what will help us to feel more alive, focused and capable.

It's being authentic and fearless in terms of doing what is best for us. We say *no* when we need to do so. We stop *doing* and start *being* to stay in balance. And we deliberately take time to feed our spirits with whatever gives us joy (aside from the temporary pleasure of the *quick fix).*

By checking in and listening to ourselves regularly, we actually create more space in our hearts to love and give to others in a healthier and more generous way.

Self-care also requires discipline and commitment. It means doing something healthy long enough to make it a habit. When work or family demands threaten to derail us, we might make a temporary adjustment to our schedule and then get right back to our plan or find a way to incorporate both (just be careful about *Superwoman Syndrome).* We could also find someone else to help out.

Sometimes it takes creativity and sometimes it means disappointing someone. However, we gain confidence as we learn we won't abandon ourselves again. The new behavior is likely to create uncomfortable feelings at first, such as guilt, anxiety, or shame. These are normal. Any breakthrough in behavior causes discomfort before we accept it as part of us.

I had a therapist who used to refer to these uncomfortable feelings as *backlash.* Knowing they are part of the growth process helps us to weather the storm rather than cause us to stifle our feelings with food or other substances.

The good news is that feelings pass and it gets easier. The initial discomfort soon gives way to greater satisfaction with ourselves and our world, which eases the need for the *quick fix.*

Affirmation:
I am authentic and fearless in terms of doing what is best for me. I care about how I feel and I treat myself with loving kindness.

New Ways to Respond
To Cravings

Getting in tune with our bodies can guide our self-care. The body is always trying to get us back into balance, so a particular craving will clue us in to what we really need. Food is really just energy. The more expansive, lighter foods like sugar or alcohol, according to a theory based on Chinese medicine, are the more *YIN* or feminine energy-type foods.

Foods gradually become more contractive as we go down the list from caffeine and sugar through milk, white flour, fruit and nuts to leafy greens and grains. The more *YANG*, masculine energy-type foods, start with root vegetables, beans, fish, and so on down to poultry, hard cheese, red meat and eggs, and finally, the most contractive—salt.

The idea is that if we eat too much of something YIN, it will create cravings for something YANG. You might try journaling to see whether this holds true for you. Frequently people will want alcohol or sweets to balance out a heavy steak dinner. By eating more in the middle of the food list we prevent the extreme cravings for foods at either end of the spectrum.

For example, the next time you crave salty foods, you can try eating some leafy greens or sea vegetables, which are high in minerals (what your body is really craving). You can try seeking a healthier version of the craving first, before reaching for the chips and dip. That way you can enjoy guilt-free satisfaction.

A craving for spicy foods may be the body's way of balancing out the more bland fatty foods that are so popular in the American diet. Spices—such as turmeric or basil, which decrease inflammation, or cinnamon, which balances blood sugar—often counteract the sluggishness that occurs from eating processed foods.

Pungent foods, like onions and garlic, enhance liver function and promote healing in the large intestine and lungs. One of my favorite pungent spices is ginger, which aids digestion. A couple of years ago I had a lingering cough and tried drinking ginger tea with lemon, cayenne pepper, cinnamon, and a half-teaspoon of raw, local honey (thought to reduce allergies). I got rid of the cough and have enjoyed this tonic many nights throughout the winter.

Cravings for sweet foods can be calmed down with lightly cooked root vegetables like carrots, onions, beets, winter squash, sweet potatoes, and yams. Even the semi-sweet vegetables like rutabagas, turnips, or parsnips are satisfying and reduce cravings for sugary, processed food.

As we gradually switch over to whole, fresh foods instead of the processed, sugary snacks, our taste buds begin to crave their fresh-tasting flavor. I often find myself savoring my salad and identifying each vegetable as I take a bite.

The fresh, crisp greens and crunchy vegetables have become the meal I crave, rather than a substitute. If I do taste something processed, such as a cake that was served at an anniversary party recently, it tastes artificial and overpoweringly sweet. It really is a matter of what we get used to, and the impact on our health is enormous.

Affirmation:
Knowledge is power and I have power over my choices today.

Healing from Cravings

I have found that what we put in our mouths either triggers addictive behavior or eases it. The same formula applies for both sugar and alcohol. Avoid the whites—sugar, bread, pasta, white potatoes, and dairy.

Cravings can further be reduced with hypoallergenic supplements like chromium, Vitamin B Complex, L-Glutamine, Lecithin, and a good high-potency multivitamin/mineral supplement with Magnesium, Carotene, and Vitamin E, according to Andrew Saul, PhD, author of *Fire Your Doctor.*

Enjoy a little cinnamon to balance blood sugar and whole, fresh foods like salads, nuts, and some fruit. Smoothies with greens, fruit and coconut water are great for starting your day.

The best way to keep cravings at bay is to eat every three to four hours, whether it is a meal or just a snack of protein and complex carbohydrates (apple and a few almonds, carrots and hummus, organic almond butter without added sugar and celery sticks). Drink plenty of fresh, filtered water throughout the day to stay hydrated.

Find some type of exercise you enjoy and get in the habit of doing it for 30 minutes at least three times a week. It boosts your endorphins and eases stress, besides keeping you fit and healthy.

Whether you are detoxifying from sugar, carbohydrates or alcohol, the more you sweat, the faster you clear out the toxins and the sooner you will feel better.

> ***Instead of the automatic reflex of opening the fridge, she has created a plan to open up other options when those feelings hit.***

Keep a notebook of your feelings and cravings along with your food log. It is vital to deciphering the connection between them. We often find a particular feeling difficult to experience, so we reach for food or alcohol or drugs to soothe it.

For example, a client recently told me that whenever she feels anger and resentment, she opens the refrigerator. Those feelings came up when she felt alone and abandoned, which are feelings she had experienced as a child. Instead of the automatic reflex of opening the fridge, she has created a plan to open up other options when those feelings hit.

I asked her to identify when the feelings came up, since awareness is the first step toward change. Next, we talked through some of those feelings to find an alternate behavior, such as writing, going for a walk, drinking a large glass of water, or promising herself that if she waited 15 minutes she could have something if she still really wanted it.

Denial that you are getting a craving often results in a slip. You are actually pushing down the feelings until they surprise you with a sudden, thoughtless urge. Instead, you want to establish and practice a different response, so the initial behavior begins to fade.

Sometimes the feelings run so deep, extra help is needed. Internal Family Systems (IFS) therapy, for example, helps you go back to the initial wound and parent yourself. It has helped me heal the young girl inside who reacted strongly every time I was triggered by a similar situation.

On a practical level, if the refrigerator is stocked with whole, fresh foods, you will not be tempted to make unhealthy choices, and eventually you lose your taste for the processed, overly sweet, fat or salty foods.

Once that stuff is out of your system, your physical cravings ease up. Author Michael Moss, who wrote *Salt, Sugar, Fat: How the Food Giants Get Us Hooked,* explains that processed foods have been designed to target our *bliss* point—that insatiable taste and texture that keeps us hooked. This is all accomplished through science and chemicals—not real food.

The rebel in me got angry when I learned how we were being manipulated to eat foods that were fattening and killing us at the same time. I vowed to avoid them, just like I quit smoking and shifted my thinking from seeing cigarettes as a crutch in times of anxiety or to relax to seeing them as disgusting cancer sticks that pollute my lungs.

Whatever it takes, we need to take back control of our health. It doesn't mean judging others who haven't reached this point yet. It just means saving ourselves and serving as an example for our families.

Affirmation:
I am free. My life freely expresses my self-love, my creativity, my unique spirit, and my purpose.

Getting through
The Crunch Times

You're probably thinking, "This is all well and good, but when that craving hits, I hit the refrigerator—period!" In that moment of struggle, you need quick tools that can help you get beyond it until the craving passes.

Researchers believe the life of a craving is about 20 minutes. If you can rely on some techniques that will get you through those crunch times, the cravings become weaker and weaker.

- Drink a large glass of water—we are often thirsty when we think we want to eat.

- Change your activity. It may be time for a break if you have been working. Take a walk or do yoga stretches—anything to break the routine.

- Ask yourself if you are really hungry or if you are bored, lonely, anxious, tired or experiencing some other unpleasant feeling that has surfaced. What is causing that feeling? Then respond to the real need.

Tell yourself you can have a small portion of what you want, but first you need to go through the steps above. Then, if you really want it, take a little bit and put the rest away. Savor it and move on.

If all else fails, get a buddy/coach you can call who can talk you through that critical period. The buddy system also works well to help you maintain good habits like walking or some other form of exercise.

Affirmation:
I don't have to do this alone. I can reach out for help whenever I need it. Support from others helps me succeed.

Ways to Combat
Social Pressure

We all need to treat ourselves gently during the early days of abstaining from our food/drink /drug of choice. It is a time of vulnerability, and a little planning and preparation will help you dodge those critical social times that encourage indulgence.

No one wants to be a hermit to eat clean and healthy—that's not the point. But early on, you may want to limit those occasions you feel are dangerous for you.

One client who had just detoxified from simple carbohydrates and sugar was invited to her in-laws' pizza party. She prepared by drinking a protein shake to fill herself up and bringing a salad to have something to eat when others were having pizza.

It turned out that salad was served as well, so she could enjoy that with everyone else and not have to respond to questions about why she wasn't having their food. The evening was a success!

I have learned over the years that people don't really care if you don't eat or drink what they do, as long as you don't spoil their enjoyment.

Simple answers like, "It doesn't sit well with me," "I'm just not hungry right now, maybe later," "I just feel like a glass of water with lime..." usually satisfy most inquiries.

Those who start to pry can be quieted with an innocuous statement like, "I'm on a health kick right now." Remember, this is your body and you don't have to please anyone but yourself.

You are also entitled to refrain from something that doesn't support you without getting the third degree. The inquiring friend or family member may just be curious or could have a problem themselves (misery loves company, you know).

Part of making different choices than others in a social situation is developing a strong sense of self.

If you hold firm in your intentions, any discomfort will quickly pass and you will become more practiced as you continue on your path. People will even get used to you making new choices.

Part of making different choices than others in a social situation is developing a strong sense of self. You become practiced at knowing what works and what doesn't for you.

Let go of trying to please others. It may cause a small flurry of resistance from them at the beginning, but your confidence will grow as you practice your own version of self-care.

Our self-care muscle needs to grow strong for us to attain our goals. It is an extension of deeply valuing ourselves and accepting our own makeup as unique. I continue to struggle with this concept. Critical voices may tell me, "You're a wimp," when I decide to stay home instead of going out.

As a highly sensitive woman, I have learned that by quieting the voice and taking an honest look at my desire, I know whether I am avoiding something or taking care of myself. If I am avoiding something, I need to ask myself what that's about, but often I am just listening to old critical voices that told me to be more like *everybody else.*

Many of us who find ourselves with cravings tend to be highly sensitive individuals. I spoke with someone recently who authored a book about parenting Indigo Children (this term was coined in the 1970s by parapsychologist and psychic Nancy Ann Tappe for children believed to possess special, unusual and sometimes supernatural traits or abilities).

This highly sensitive friend asked me whether I thought the tendency toward addiction or recurrent cravings was a soul-based problem. Actually, I think it is both soul- and genetics-based.

The right environmental triggers have to be present to turn on the gene, but it is also about filling a hole inside. By whatever spiritual means resonates with you, that hole needs to be filled up.

No one else can do it for you. For me, it was a spiritual awakening that deepened over time. I suggest you explore ways to connect to a higher power/Source/God. It helps you feel connected and loved, while you face your fears, feelings and move through to the other side of your struggle where your true inner peace resides.

Affirmation:
The only person I need to please is myself. The more I practice loving myself, the deeper my capacity to love others.

What's in Your Future?
A Case Study

Let's contrast the lives of two adults married to each other named Jack and Janet. Jack is 35 and busy climbing the corporate ladder. He has a wife and two children, ages 4 and 6. Jack is on the go, traveling to different cities during the week and eating in restaurants three to five days a week.

His job requires plenty of wining and dining, so Jack is beginning to show a bit of a paunch over his belt. He works out sporadically. He starts out with good intentions but gets easily derailed by deadlines and the other demands of an overburdened schedule.

Jack's doctor tells him his HDL cholesterol levels are low, his triglycerides are high, and he has developed high blood pressure. He is actually pre-diabetic or has what is known as metabolic syndrome. By the way, Jack's dad is also diabetic, and if he keeps going like this, within 10 years Jack will have full-blown diabetes himself.

Meanwhile, Jack's wife, Janet, is managing the household and raising their two small children. She prepares her meals most days and walks the dog for about a half hour every day. Janet is also 35.

Life is hectic, but Janet wants her children to develop healthy eating habits, so meals are usually made from fresh vegetables, lean meat, salads, beans, and whole grains.

She gives the children apples and almonds or carrots and hummus for snacks. Janet has a few close friends she stays in contact with, and her family lives nearby.

It doesn't take much thought to see who is likely to live a healthier, longer life. Do you know what is happening to each of them on the inside, though?

Jack's diet of processed, sugar-laden foods throws off the balance of minerals in his body. The imbalance of minerals then affects the ability of the body's enzymes to metabolize food.

In fact, according to author Nancy Appleton, "When you eat sugar, any food that is in the stomach at the time will become the food to which you can become allergic."

The person who develops allergies exhausts their immune system, and the body becomes susceptible to other diseases. Now the degenerative process has begun. If he keeps on going the way he is living now, by the time Jack is 40, he probably won't feel right most of the time.

When we develop food allergies, we also develop cravings, which, in turn, lead to addictions and overeating.

The damage from sugar is interfering with his metabolic processes, and he could have one or more of the following conditions: Headaches, constipation, bloating, tooth decay, psoriasis, canker sores, and candida.

He'll probably be about 10 pounds heavier, too. When we develop food allergies, we also develop cravings, which, in turn, lead to addictions and overeating.

As time goes on, Jack may develop gallstones, arthritis, asthma, hypoglycemia, inflammatory bowel disease, diabetes or cancer. All it takes for Jack to reverse this process is a decision to stop upsetting his mineral balance with sugar.

Whether he continues his high-pressure job or not will have an impact, but what he eats and how he cares for his body in terms of exercise and rest will mediate the stress.

Meanwhile, Janet has joined a yoga class and meditates in the morning when the house is quiet. She has started her own business teaching others to make greeting cards, which gives her the creative outlet she needs.

Janet's diet has become both gluten and sugar-free, and she eats primarily fish and white meat. At 40, her friends tell her she looks a good five years younger, and she feels fantastic. Her body is in homeostasis metabolically.

When Janet gets a craving, it's her body's way of telling her what it needs, from greens to beans to fruit to nuts. This is because her body is no longer getting false signals from too much fat, salt, or sugar. Barring any unforeseen accidents, Janet will continue to enjoy a long, healthy, and active life.

Affirmation:
I am committed to taking the steps that will help me live a long, active joyful life.

Start Right Now: Freedom is Within Reach

I know a long, healthy, active life is the goal of many of us who are at various stages of health. Unfortunately, it often takes some sort of scare to get us moving in the right direction.

If you make up your mind to start now, much of the damage done can be reversed by a healthy way of eating, elimination of foods that cause cravings, and a lifestyle that honors what we need.

(Visit my website for a checklist of action steps to get you started: sherylturgeon.com/cravings-your-guide-to-freedom/cravings-bonuses/).

If you make up your mind to start now, much of the damage done can be reversed by a healthy way of eating, elimination of foods that cause cravings, and a lifestyle that honors what we need.

Just remember, while your future is in your hands, you don't have to do it alone. You have some great resources out there, and I want to give you the help that was given to me when I needed it. Starting today you can give yourself more life choices and finally break free of the cravings, patterns and habits that no longer work for you.

To connect with me, just go to my website (SheryTurgeon.com) and schedule a brief time to chat. We'll talk about where you're concerned and how you're feeling, so we can discover the best options to help you.

I have been at this for quite a while and I still have my occasional slips. I realized long ago that gluten and dairy were toxic to me.

Yet, now and then I seem to have to give it another try. I think of it as experimenting to see if I really am still sensitive to the stuff. Sure enough, every time I experiment, I find out that *yes, I really am! Enough already!*

I'm passionate about helping you strengthen that confidence-building muscle. It will take you far in so many ways, from healing cravings to following your dreams!

We need to be aware that one slip can unravel how far we've come once we've eliminated our cravings. When you notice the craving reawakening, see it as a *red flag*. It's time to take extra measures to get that food out of your diet again using the guidelines on my website: http://sherylturgeon.com/cravings-your-guide-to-freedom/cravings-bonuses/.

The key is to encourage—not berate—ourselves. I'm passionate about helping you strengthen that confidence-building muscle. It will take you far in so many ways, from healing cravings to following your dreams!

Ask questions. When I find myself making unhealthy choices, I try to pay attention to what's really going on. Do I need more stimulation? Am I over-stimulated? Do I feel hungry, angry, lonely, or tired?

Did I simply act impulsively and forget? That is a tough one and can happen before we know it, which is why we build in new habits to keep automatic impulses at bay.

If the craving is for something deadly for you like alcohol or drugs, a slip may not allow another chance. For most, the craving is more about sweets and carbohydrates. They won't kill us—at least not quickly—but they can lead to so many deadly degenerative diseases, it's really not worth the risk.

Stay in the present moment as much as you can, so you are aware of how you're feeling. Then get what you really need instead of finding an unhealthy substitute.

It's a messy, sometimes painful journey, but the other side offers freedom, vitality, better moods, improvement of chronic conditions, your ideal weight, and relief at last from that incessant and agonizing merry-go-round.

You will also come to know yourself much better during the process, which can have a profound impact on your life.

Affirmation:
Now that I know what does and doesn't work for me, I honor my body by making choices that make me feel good.

Are You Ready to Take The First Step?

I wish you joy, peace, and freedom from cravings, plus an outstretched hand from someone who's been there... just grab onto some of my hope until you create your own.

I was once told that adult children of alcoholics needed every resource they could get to heal from the effects of their childhood environment.

I think the wounds we all carry manifest in our relationships, our cravings, and our patterns that block us from who we really want to be—I'll bet you know what they are for you.

Healing is about embracing new behaviors and shifting your mindset. It is much bigger than the symptom of a craving. If you are really ready to say *"Enough!"* to those old ways, you are ready for a transformation that will uplift you on every level of your being. That's what I most want for you—to see you shed your cocoon and spread your wings to thrive in a life that becomes even greater than you've imagined.

Cravings are merely the window through which you will soar to your next evolution. They are pestering you now for a reason and the universe is prodding you to rise to the occasion.

Are you ready to accept the challenge? You only need to ask and you'll get the help you need to find your way out... Reach now for the grander view and the freedom to be you!

Affirmation:
I embrace the new me, even when it feels uncomfortable.

Glossary

Adenosine Triphosphate (ATP): Our cells' energy source. It transports chemical energy within cells for metabolism.

Antigen: A substance that stimulates the production of an antibody when introduced into the body. *Antigens* include toxins, bacteria, viruses, and other foreign substances.

Candida: A type of yeast, it is only a problem if it is the dominant bacteria in our intestines. It's also the most common condition caused by a sugary and starchy diet, because it lives off sugar. This means any sugar you eat feeds it. Since all starches get broken down as sugar, grains, sugary fruit, starchy vegetables and lactose (sugar in milk) feed Candida.

DHEA: Dehydroepiandrosterone (DHEA) is a hormone that comes from the adrenal gland. It is also made in the brain. DHEA leads to the production of androgens and estrogens (male and female sex hormones). DHEA levels in the body begin to decrease after age 30. Levels decrease more quickly in women. It is known to reduce aging and stress.

Dysbiosis: An imbalance in gut bacteria. It can result from a deficiency of good bacteria or an overgrowth of harmful organisms. In either case, organisms that are not usually predominant in the intestines, such as unfriendly bacteria, yeast (candida) and protozoa, actually induce disease by altering nutrition patterns in the body.

Fructose: A simple sugar like glucose. The main difference is that fructose is metabolized by the liver, while glucose is metabolized by insulin from the pancreas.

The key here is that while every cell in the body can use glucose, the liver is the only organ that can metabolize fructose in significant amounts. When people eat a diet that is high in calories and fructose, the liver gets overloaded and starts turning the fructose into fat.

Scientists believe that excess fructose consumption in processed foods may be a key driver of many of the most serious diseases today, including obesity, type II diabetes, heart disease and even cancer.

Grehlin: A hormone that increases appetite, and also plays a role in body weight. It is produced and released mainly by the stomach with small amounts also released by the small intestine, pancreas and brain. Grehlin is called the *hunger hormone* because it stimulates appetite, increases food intake and promotes fat storage.

High Fructose Corn Syrup: An artificially manufactured sweetener made from corn that has been added to simple carbohydrates to prolong shelf-life and inexpensively increase the sweetness of a product. The composition is 42 percent or 55 percent fructose, *with the remaining sugars being primarily glucose and higher sugars.*

Internal Family Systems Therapy: A therapy developed by Richard C. Schwartz, PhD., aimed at healing wounds associated with traumatic situations can be applied in family, couple, and individual situations. A person progresses on their own healing path according to their unique design without external urgency or persuasion.

IgA Antibodies: Immunoglobulin A (also referred to as sIgA) is an antibody that plays a critical role in mucosal immunity. More IgA is produced in mucosal linings than all other types of antibody combined. IgA antibodies are found in areas of the body such the nose, breathing passages, digestive tract, ears, eyes, and vagina.

IgG Antibodies: Immunoglobulin G (IgG), the most abundant type of antibody, is found in all body fluids and protects against bacterial and viral infections.

Leptin: A hormone that plays a crucial role in appetite and weight control. It crosses the blood-brain barrier and binds to receptors in the appetite center in the brain, regulating brain cells that tell you how much to eat. It also increases sympathetic nervous system activity, which stimulates fatty tissue to burn energy.

Metabolic Syndrome: Often identified by a pear-shaped figure, metabolic syndrome is a cluster of conditions — increased blood pressure, a high blood sugar level, excess body fat around the waist and abnormal cholesterol levels — that occur together, increasing your risk of heart disease, stroke and diabetes.

NSAIDs: Non-steroidal anti-inflammatory drugs that reduce inflammation, pain, and fever. However, they interfere with the production of prostaglandins that protect the stomach and support platelets and blood clotting, so NSAIDs can cause ulcers in the stomach and promote bleeding.

Transient Global Amnesia: A sudden, temporary episode of memory loss that can't be attributed to a more common neurological condition, such as epilepsy or stroke. Risk is higher in patients with migraines.

Triglycerides: A type of fat found in your blood. Your body uses them for energy. You need some *triglycerides* for good health. But high *triglycerides* might raise your risk of heart disease and may be a sign of metabolic syndrome.

Bonuses and Resources

Please go to:

www.sherylturgeon.com/cravings-your-guide-to-freedom/cravings-bonuses/
to access the following bonus downloadable documents:

Action Steps for Great Health

Affirmations

Amazing Secrets of Self Care

Cravings Strategies That Work

Food and Feelings Awareness Journal

Sumptuous Sugar Free Snack Ideas

Testing for Food Sensitivities

To learn more about my programs, visit:

www.sherylturgeon.com/
    coaching-programs/

Ways to connect with me.

Free Chat Session:
www.meetme.so/SherylTurgeon

Email:
www.sherylturgeon.com/
    contact-sheryl-turgeon/

Facebook Page:
www.facebook.com/SherylTurgeonBiz

Facebook Group:
www.facebook.com/groups/
    HSWcommunity

About The Author

It's been over eight years since Sheryl left her long-term position as CEO of a Community Health Center and launched her business coaching highly sensitive women as an Integrative Health Coach.

Sheryl discovered how sensitivities affected her and others on a physical, emotional and mental level. Getting healthy meant a transformational shift that requires creating balance in all aspects of their lives.

Her exploration into the effects of various foods on each client led her to create a program to help eliminate food sensitivities and help women discover the best food for them.

Sheryl is passionate about helping women reach and maintain their ideal weight, nourish their bodies and spirits with courageous self-care, and finding and following their passion to share their unique gifts with the world.

She has been reaching out through her video and TV show, **_Living Healthy_**, along with sharing alternative health concepts as a Boston radio show host.

A former columnist and now, author of the book, **_Cravings! Your Guide to Freedom from the Agonizing Urge to Splurge,_** Sheryl uses her journalism background to weave in personal stories, tips and tools, and to simplify the science of what drives cravings.

To read more about Sheryl Turgeon and her expertise or hire her for your next event, go to her website at:

www.SherylTurgeon.com.

Made in the USA
Middletown, DE
15 May 2016